PRACTICAL BOOK OF PHARMACEUTICS I

B.PHARM SEMESTER I (AS PER LATEST SYLLABUS PRESCRIBED BY P.C.I)

DR. SHIKHA BAGHEL CHAUHAN

Contents

Preface

Pharmaceutics 1 Practical Book- B. Pharm 1st Year 1st Semester Book

(As per latest PCI Regulations).

The Pharmaceutics Practical Book is designed for B. Pharmacy 1st Sem (First year) students and is strictly as per the Pharmacy Council of India (PCI) regulations.

Pharmaceutics 1 Book aims to impart a fundamental knowledge on the preparatory Pharmacy with arts and science of preparing the different conventional dosage forms. The content of this practical manual is prepared according to the revised syllabus given by PCI (Pharmacy Council of India) and provides students practical knowledge about pharmaceutics I.

This manual is incorporated with all the conventional dosage form preparations such as solutions, syrups, elixir, linctus, emulsions, suspensions etc. core concepts and underlying principles has been discussed, method of preparation of all the formulations are explained thoroughly.

This course is designed to impart a fundamental knowledge on the preparatory

pharmacy with arts and science of preparing the different conventional dosage forms.

Upon completion of this course the student should be able to:

? Know the history of profession of pharmacy

? Understand the basics of different dosage forms, pharmaceutical incompatibilities and pharmaceutical calculations.

? Understand the professional way of handling the prescription

? Preparation of various conventional dosage forms

The emphasis is given to the theory/ principle involved in each formulation of Pharmaceutics 1. Thus, the simplicity and illustrative presentation of the Pharmaceutics book 1st Semester will assist the students to understand the basics of different dosage.

This book will be highly useful by B. Pharmacy 1st Semester students.

Acknowledgements

Acknowledgements

It is our immense pleasure to publish and present Practical Book of Pharmaceutics I to the pharmaceutical sciences students, teachers, and research scholars.

Any successful outcome is not an individual effort, but it is a joint venture of many people who put in their mind and soul for the completion of the work.

I would like to acknowledge the extraordinary debt I owe to my dear students Vinamra, Vinita and Shallu Sharma. *I would never have been able, to complete this book without their support and motivation.*

I am pleased to express my deep sense of gratitude towards my parents for their constant encouragement and motivation to transform my teachings in the form of a user-friendly book for the students.

I hope this book will help the students in understanding the core concepts of subject and develop deep understanding of subject.

The readers of this book are requested to present their reviews and suggestions which will be highly appreciated and accepted by the authors. Constructive suggestions, comments and criticism on the subject matter of the book will be gratefully acknowledged, as they will certainly help to improve future editions of the book.

CHAPTER ONE

EXPERIMENT 1

AIM: To study various parts of a prescription along with various Latin terms used in prescription and to study the various guidelines for the preparation of pharmaceutical labels.

THEORY:

Prescription is an order written by a physician, dentist, or any other medical practitioner to the pharmacist to compound & dispense a specific medication for individual patient. It is a direct link between the physician, pharmacist & the patient.

Prescription is accompanied by directions for the pharmacist & for the patient. It has same codes as:

1. For adults.
2. Special Instructions for Particular Types of Products
3. Pressurized inhalations
4. Capsules
5. Creams
6. Dusting powder
7. Emulsions
8. Enemas
9. Eye drops
10. Gargles and mouthwashes
11. Gels
12. Linctus
13. Ointments, paints & pastes
14. Tablets
15. Chewable tablets
16. Sustained release/enteric coated tablet
17. J for a juvenile under 16 years of age.
18. Y for a child under 10 years of age
19. O for oral contraception.

A prescription has various parts:

Heading: It comprises the date & personal information (like age, sex, address, name) of the patient.

Body

Body comprises of three main parts :

a. <u>Superscription:</u> It mainly comprises of the term 'Rx' which is an abbreviation for Latin word "recipere" or "recipe" which means "take, thou". This is said to designate 'Jupiter, the God of Healing.

b. <u>Inscription:</u> It is the main part of prescription that contains the name & quantity of prescribed medicines and the manner in which they should be taken.

c. <u>Subscription:</u> It comprises of the instructions for the pharmacist which includes:

I. Type of dosage to be prepared.
II. No. of dosages to be dispensed.

Closing- It comprises of the signature of the physician. The address & registration number should be written in case of dangerous drugs.

SAMPLE PREPARATION:

BEST HOSPITAL

100W, MAIN, HOME TOWN, USA, PH:12345554321

NAME: ____________ DATE: ____________

ADDRESS: ____________ AGE: ____________

RX "GNE FULL DIRECTIONS FOR USE

REFILLS: 0-1-2-3-4-5- ________

____
SIGNATURE OF PRESCRIBER

DEA # ____________

LABEL UNLESS CHECKED HERE ☐

____
NAME (PRINTED)

GENERIC SUBSTITUTION UNLESS CHECKED HERE ☐

U.S. DEPARTMENT OF HEALTH AND HUMAN SERVICES, PUBLIC HEALTH SERVICES

Sample Prescription

Latin terms are used while writing the prescription as latin is more concise tha other language.
Latin is universally understood among medical professionals.
Latin terms are used as:

1. Doctors' shorthand for communicating with the pharmacist.
2. Doctor advice the medication protocol in the subscription of the prescription.
3. It indicates the route of medication as well as dispensing method.

Labelling: label means display of printed information which is securely affixed to the containers and primary packaging containing the medicines. A label should provide the patient with all the necessary information for appropriate use of medicines like

A. General labelling requirements
B. Cautionary & advisory labels

C. Special instructions for different types of products

D. Accurate, legible, intelligible, adequate & relevant information should be provided.

A label is required to distinguish the product from products of other brands It is a legal requirement to provide a label.

General Labelling Requirements are:

a. Name of the preparation.

b. Strength & dosage form.

c. Quantity

d. Instructions for use

e. Precautions & warnings

f. Registration number of the company

g. Batch number

h. Manufacturing & expiry dates.

I. Price

j. Storage instructions

k. Name & address of the pharmaceutical company dispensing the drug.

SAMPLE LABEL:

Rx

MONTELUKAST SODIUM TABLETS IP 10MG

MONTAIR-10

EACH FILM- COATED TABLET
CONTAINS MONTELUKAST
SODIUM IP EQUIVALENT TO
MONTELUKAST.............10MG

COLOURS: TITANIUM DIOXIDE AND YELLOW OXIDE OF IRON

DOSAGE: AS DIRECTED BY THE PHYSICIAN

MFG BY: CIPLA LTD. CIPLA
KUMREK, RANGO, SIKKIM, 737132, INDIA

21047064

Storage below 30°C

Protect from light and moisture

Schedule H Drug Warning:
To be sold by retail on the prescription of a registered medical practitioner only.

M.L. M/447/2007

BATCH NO. E20138, **MFD.**JAN 2020

EXP. DEC2021

MRP FOR 15 TABS. RS. 239.25 INCL. OF ALL TAXES

SAMPLE LABEL

Cautionary & Advisory Labels:

- For external use only (Ointments, creams, dusting powders, gels etc.)
- Not to be taken orally (For nasal, rectal, vaginal use)
- Not to be swallowed in large amounts (For mouth washes, gargles)
- Keep out of reach of children
- For animal treatment only
- **Drowsiness Warnings:**

  Drowsiness, dizziness, blurred vision, or difficulty in concentrating
- **For children's medicines:** Warning. May cause drowsiness
- Some medicines make patients drowsier especially when consuming alcohol.
- Hypnotics used as sleep aids taken at bedtime may cause drowsiness persisting the next day.

- Potential interactions with food or drink
- Products liable to cause GIT irritation
- Better desorption with food.
- Same medicines have improved desorption without food (oral antibiotics)
- Exert effect on GIT prior to food.
- Potentials interactions with other medicines
- The problem can be avoided by giving incompatible preparations 2 hrs apart.
- special dosage Instruction
- Special method of administration
- Cautions in use

Direction for external use depicted on various labels:

FOR EXTERNAL USE ONLY

THIS MEDICINE MAY CAUSE DROWSINESS AND MAY INCREASE TH EFFECTS OF ALCOHOL.

IF AFFECTED, DONOT DRIVE OR OPERATE MACHINERY.

WARNING- MAY CAUSE DROWSINESS

THIS PREPARATION IS TO AID SLEEP. DROWSINESS MAY CONTINUE THE FOLLOWING DAY. IF AFFECTED, DONOT DRIVE OR OPERATE MACHINERY. AVOID ALCOHOL

THIS MEDICINE MAY AFFECT MENTAL ALERTNESS OR COORDINATION. IF AFFECTED, DONOT DRIVE VEHICLE OR OPERATE MACHINERY.

.... WITH OR AFTER FOOD

PRESSURIZED CONTAINER, KEEP AWAY FROM HEAT SOURCE INCLUDING THE SUN. DONOT PUNCTURE OR BURN EVEN WHEN EMPTY. SHAKE BEFORE USING

TAKE HALF TO ONE HOUR BEFOR FOOD OR EMPTY STOMACH

AVOID EXPOSURE OF SKIN TO DIRECT SUNLIGHT

THIS PREPARATION MAY COLOUR THE URINE OR STOOL

DONOT TAKE IRON, MILK, OR INDIGESTION REMEDIES AT SAME TIME OF THE DAY AS THIS MEDICINE

DONOT STOP TAKING THIS MEDICINE EXPCEPT ON YOUR DOCTOR'S ADVICE

TAKE AT REGULAR INTERVALS. COMPLETE THE PRESCRIBED COURSE UNLESS OTHERWISE DIRECTED.

DISSOLVE OR MIX WITH WATER BEFORE TAKING

DISSOLVE UNDER THE TONGUE

.... WITH PLENTY OF WATER

.... SWALLOW WHOLE NOT CHEWED

Direction for external use

Special Instructions for Particular Types of Products

- Pressurized inhalations
- Capsules
- Creams
- Dusting powder
- Emulsions
- Enemas
- Eye drops
- Gargles and mouthwashes
- Gels
- Linctus
- Ointments, paints & pastes
- Tablets
- Chewable tablets
- Sustained release/enteric coated tablet\

SWALLOW WHOLE WITH A DRAUGHT OF WATER

STORE IN COOL PLACE BUT DONOT FREEZE

FOR EXTERNAL USE ONLY

NOT TO BE APPLIED TO OPEN WOUNDS OR WEEPING SURFACES

SHAKE THE BOTTLE

FOR RECTAL USE ONLY

SHAKE BEFORE USE

NOT TO BE SWALLOWED IN LARGE AMOUNT

FOR EXTERNAL USE ONLY

TO BE SIPPED AND SWALLOWED SLOWLY WITHOUT THE ADDITION OF WATER

FOR EXTERNAL USE ONLY

DISSOLVE OR DISPENSE IN WATER BEFORE TAKING

CHEW BEFORE SWALLOWING

DONOT CHEW BEFORE SWALLOWING

Special Instructions for Particular Types of Products

CONCLUSION

Various parts of prescription along with various Latin terms used in prescription and guidelines for the preparation of pharmaceutical labels were studied.

CHAPTER TWO

EXPERIMENT 2

AIM- To prepare and dispense simple syrup IP.

MATERIAL REQUIRED- Sucrose, beaker, stirrer, spatula, measuring cylinder & purified water.

THEORY-

Syrups are sweetened, viscous, concentrated solutions of sucrose or other sugars in water or any other suitable aqueous vehicles. A simple syrup contains only sugar (sucrose) & purified water, syrup containing pleasantly flavoured substances are known as flavoured syrups which can be syrups to which therapeutic compounds are added are called medicinal syrups. Simple or flavouring syrups are added to mask the disagreeable taste of the drug. A preservative should be added to the syrup if sucrose concentration is less than 85% w/v.

A simple syrup can have different concentrations as per different pharmacopoeias:

1. IP- 66.7% w/w
2. USP- 85% w/w
3. BP- 85% w/w

Rx

NOT FOR DIABETIC PATIENTS

SIMPLE SYRUP IP 100ml

SUGAR SYRUP 66.7

1000ml of syrup contains 667gm of sucrose

COLOUR: COLOURLESS

DOSAGE: AS DIRECTED BY PHYSICIAN

INGREDIENTS: SUCROSE (33.35gm),

DISTILLED WATER (50ml or q.s.)

MFD. BY-

V.G. PHARMA

320, SOLAN INDUSTRIAL AREA,
HIMACHAL PRADESH, INDIA

REG NO.-1247983

B. NO- 73EF20T

EXP- 24/03/2022

MFD- 15/09/2020

MRP- Rs. 40.00

STORE AT A TEMPERATURE NOT EXCEEDING 25°C

Simple syrup Label

PROCEDURE-

- Add water to sucrose in a beaker and heat on water bath until sucrose dissolves. Add sufficient boiling water to produce the final volume.
- Filter hot syrup through cotton wool.
- Cool the syrup and preservative for stability.

Sr. No.	INGREDIENTS	QUANTITY PRESCRIBED	QUANTITY TAKEN
1.	Sucrose	667gm	33.35gm
2.	Distilled water	1000ml	50ml

Simple syrup Composition

RESULT

50 ml of simple syrup was prepared and dispensed.

STORAGE

Store in tightly closed container at cool temperature not exceeding 25°C in dark place.

PRECAUTIONS

- Boiling water should be handled with care.
- Ensure zero reading on weighing scale before weighing anything.

VIVA QUESTIONS

1. *Define syrups.*
2. *What is concentration of sugar used in simple syrup I.P. and why?*
3. *What are medicated and flavoured syrups?*
4. *What are general conditions for storage of syrups?*
5. *What is the use of simple syrup I.P.?*
6. *How do you prepare simple syrup I.P?*
7. *Give pharmaceutical applications of simple syrup I.P.*

CHAPTER THREE

EXPERIMENT 3

AIM : To prepared and dispense 50 ml of compound ferrous sulphate syrup I.P.

MATERIAL REQUIRED

Ferrous sulphate ($FeSo_4$), citric acid, peppermint spirit, sucrose, water, beaker, glass rod and measuring cylinder.

THEORY

Syrups are sweetened, viscous, concentrated solutions of sucrose or other sugars in water or any other suitable aqueous vehicles.

Ferrous sulphate syrup is an iron supplement used to treat or prevent low blood levels of iron (caused by anaemia or pregnancy). Iron is an important mineral that helps producing RBCs, it is a hematinic (nutrient required for producing RBCs).

Ferrous sulphate is used as a source of iron.

Citric acid is used to stabilise $FeSo_4$ against oxidation to more toxic Fe (111) form.

Peppermint oil is used by making a spirit out of it by mixing it with ethanol. It is used as flavouring agent.

Sucrose is used as a sweetening agent.

Fe+ 2H3PO4------- Fe (H2P04)2+ H2O

FERROUS SULPHATE SYRUP IP 50ml

FERROMATINIC SYRUP

EACH 5ml CONTAINS 0.2g W/V FERROUS SULPHATE

INGREDIENTS: FERROUS SULPHATE (2g), CITRIC ACID (0.105g), PEPPERMINT SPIRIT (0.1ml), SUCROSE (41.25g), PURIFIED WATER (50ml or q.s.)

DOSAGE: AS DIRECTED BY PHYSICIAN

STORAGE: STORE PROTECTED FROM LIGHT IN ORIGINAL CONTAINER

MFD BY-

VG PHARMA

320, SOLAN INDUSTRIAL AREA, HIMACHAL PRADESH, INDIA

REG NO- 1247892

B. NO.- ZPM842X

MFG.D- 28/09/2022

EXP.D- 29/09/2022

MRP- Rs.76.00

INCL. ALL TAXES

Ferrous sulphate syrup Label

PROCEDURE-

1. Dissolve ferrous sulphate, citric acid, peppermint spirit and sucrose in sufficient quantity of water.
2. Filter the solution.
3. Add purified water to make up the quantity to 50 ml.

S No.	INGREDIENTS	QUANITITY PRESCRIBED	QUANTITY USED
1.	Ferrous sulphate	40g	2g
2.	Citric acid	2.1g	0.105g
3.	Peppermint spirit	2ml	0.1ml
4.	sucrose	825g	41.25g
5.	Purified water	1000ml	50ml

Ferrous sulphate syrup Composition

DOSE

Each 5ml contains 0.2g w/v of ferrous sulphate

DIRECTION

For internal use only.

USE

Hematinic

STORAGE

It should be stored in amber coloured bottles, avoid direct sunlight and store at room temperature.

RESULT

50 ml of ferrous sulphate was prepared and dispensed.

VIVA- QUESTIONS

1. ***What is synonym for compound ferrous sulphate syrup I.P.?***
2. ***What is the use of compound ferrous sulphate syrup I.P.?***
3. ***What is the purpose of adding flavour ants and colourants in syrups?***
4. ***Name some artificial sweeteners.***
5. ***What are storage conditions for compound ferrous sulphate syrup I.P.?***
6. ***What is use of compound ferrous sulphate syrup I.P.?***
7. ***What is method of preparation for compound ferrous sulphate syrup I.P.?***

CHAPTER FOUR

EXPERIMENT 4

AIM : To Prepare and Dispense 30ml of Paediatric Paracetamol Elixir B.P.

MATERIAL REQUIRED- Paracetamol, sugar syrup, beaker, glass rod and measuring cylinder, amaranth solution, chloroform spirit, concentrated raspberry juice, propylene glycol, invert syrup, glycerol etc.

FORMULA

INGREDIENTS	STANDARD FORMULA	WORKING FORMULA	ROLE OF INGREDIENTS
Paracetamol	24g	0.72g	Analgesic and antipyretic
Amaranth solution	2ml	0.006ml	Colouring agent
Chloroform spirit	20ml	0.6 ml	Flavouring agent
Concentrated raspberry juice	25ml	0.75ml	Colouring and flavouring agent
Alcohol	100ml	3ml	Co- solvent
Propylene glycol	100ml	3ml	Co- solvent
Invert sugar	275ml	8.25ml	Sweetening agent
Glycerol q.s. to produce	1000ml	30ml	vehicle

Paediatric Paracetamol Elixir Composition

THEORY

Syrups are sweetened, viscous, concentrated solutions of sucrose or other sugars in water or any other suitable aqueous vehicle.

In paracetamol podiatric syrup, paracetamol acts as an antipyretic, analgesic, and sugar syrup acts as flavoured vehicles.

Antipyretics: A substance that reduces fever. Antipyretics cause the hypothalamus to override a prostaglandin induced increase in temperature. The body then works to lower the temperature, which results in a reduction in fever.

Analgesic: Medicines that are used to relieve pain. They are also known as painkiller or pain relievers. They provide relief as pain without putting us to sleep or making us lose consciousness.

Amaranth solution is used as colouring agent.

Chloroform spirit is used as flavouring agent, concentrated raspberry juice is used as colouring and flavouring agent.

Invert syrup and **glycerol** are sweeting agent and vehicles.

Rx

PARACETAMOL PAEDIATRIC SYRUP IP 30ml

BABYMOL SYPRUP

Each 5ml contains 125mg of paracetamol

DOSAGE: AS DIRECTED BY PAEDIATRICIAN

STORE IN WELL CLOSED CONTAINER IN A COOL PLACE

MFD BY-	**B. NO**- 847PQ2
VG PHARMA	**MFD. D**- 22/09/2020
320, SOLAN INDUSTRIAL AREA, HIMACHAL PRADESH, INDIA	**EXP. D**- 21/09/2022
REG NO- 1247892	**MRP**- Rs. 60.00
	INCL. ALL TAXES

INGREDIENTS- Paracetamol (0.075gm), Sucrose (20.01gm), Distilled Water (30ml, q.s.), Preservatives (q.s.)

Paediatric Paracetamol Elixir Label

PROCEDURE

1. Dissolve weighed amount of paracetamol in a mixture of the alcohol and the chloroform spirit.
2. Dilute the raspberry juice with invert syrup, amaranth solution, propylene glycol and glycerol.
3. Add the solution prepared in the above prepared mixture of paracetamol and mix well.
4. Transfer to a measuring cylinder and adjust to the final volume with glycerol.
5. Transfer contents to the amber coloure3de narrow mouth plastic or glass bottle and close the container tightly with screw cap, polish, and label.

CATEGORY
To treat mild to moderate pain as anti- pyretic and in post immunisation pyrexia.
DOSE
Each 5ml contains 125 mg of paracetamol.
DIRECTION
Shake the bottle well before use for at least 10 secs,For internal use only.
USE
Antipyretic and analgesic.
STORAGE
Store in a well closed container in a cool place.

CONTRAINDICATIONS

Hypersensitivity to paracetamol and other constituents.

RESULT

The paracetamol paediatric syrup was prepared and dispense.

VIVA- QUESTIONS

1. ***What are elixirs?***
2. ***What are types of elixirs?***
3. ***What are directions for use of paediatric paracetamol elixir?***
4. ***Define analgesic and antipyretics.***
5. ***What are the uses of paediatric paracetamol elixir?***
6. ***Why paediatric syrups are formulated as flavoured syrups containing little or no alcohol?***
7. ***What is use of invert sugar and glycerol in paediatric paracetamol elixir?***

CHAPTER FIVE

EXPERIMENT 5

AIM : To Prepare and dispense Piperazine Citrate Elixir.

MATERIAL REQUIRED- Beaker, glass rod, glass funnel, glass bottle, Piperazine citrate BPC, Peppermint oil, glycerine, purified water etc.

FORMULA-

INGREDIENTS	QUANTITY USED
Piperazine citrate	180gm
Chloroform Spirit	5ml
Glycerine	100ml
Orange oil	0.25ml
Syrup	500ml
Purified water	q.s. or 1000ml

Piperazine Citrate Elixir Composition

THEORY-

Piperazine citrate is used for pinworm infections, threadworm infections, roundworm infections and other conditions. This formulation is an oral solution containing 15.3 to 17.7 w/v of piperazine citrate as an active ingredient in a suitable flavoured vehicle. Piperazine is rapidly absorbed from the gastrointestinal tract, it is almost white or granular, crystalline powder that melts at about 190˚C.

Elixirs are clear, liquid, oral preparations of potent drugs (like antibiotics, antihistaminic, sedatives, etc.) or unpalatable drugs. They are pleasantly flavoured and usually attractively coloured.

In this elixirs Propylene glycol, ethanol, and glycerol these are all acts a vehicle and co-solvent to increase the solubility of poorly soluble ingredients.

Chloroform spirit acts as a preservative.

Invert syrup acts as a sweetening agent.

The Percentage of alcohol varies from 4 to 40 %.

Piperazine Citrate Elixir BPC

FORMULA- Piperazine citrate (180gm), Chloroform Spirit (5ml), Glycerine (100ml), Orange oil (0.25ml), Syrup (500ml), Purified water (q.s. or 1000ml)

USES- Anti-helminthic

STORAGE- Stored in a well closed container at a temperature not exceeding 25°C.

B. NO.- XP24322

MFG.D- 22/09/2022

EXP.D- 21/09/2022

MRP- Rs.100.00

INCL. ALL TAXES

MFG- VG PHARMA, 320, SOLAN INDUSTRIAL AREA, HIMACHAL PRADESH, INDIA

REG NO- 1247892

Piperazine Citrate Elixir Sample Label

PROCEDURE

1. Piperazine citrate is dissolved in small amount of purified water.
2. Orange oil, glycerine, syrup, and chloroform spirit is mixed.
3. Sufficient volume is added to produce the final volume.

USES

Anthelmintic

DOSE

9 to 12 months: 2.5ml
2 to 3 years: 5ml
4 to 6 years: 7.5ml
7 to 12 years: 10ml

STORAGE

Stored in a well closed container at a temperature not exceeding 25°C.

RESULT

Piperazine Citrate Elixir BPC was successfully prepared and dispensed.

VIVA QUESTIONS

1. *What are the types of elixirs?*
2. *How are elixirs made clear?*
3. *Name some marketed formulations of elixirs.*
4. *What is use of piperazine citrate elixir syrup?*
5. *Name and manufacture any piperazine citrate elixir syrup.*
6. *What is role of chloroform is piperazine citrate elixir syrup?*
7. *What dose of piperazine citrate elixir syrup is recommended?*
8. *What is strength of piperazine citrate elixir syrup?*
9. *What types of infections are treated by piperazine citrate elixir syrup?*

10. ***What is important direction of use for piperazine citrate elixir syrup?***

CHAPTER SIX

EXPERIMENT 6

AIM- To Prepare and dispense Terpin Hydrate Linctus.

MATERIAL REQUIRED - Beaker, glass rod, glass funnel, terpin hydrate, orange oil, glycerine, alcohol, syrup, purified water

FORMULA

INGREDIENTS	QUANTITY USED	ROLE OF INGREDIENTS
Terpin hydrate	50gm	Expectorant
Orange oil	0.2ml	Flavouring agent
Glycerine	400ml	Demulcent
Alcohol	425ml	Solublizer
Syrup	100ml	Sweetening agent
Purified water	q.s. or 1000ml	Vehicle

Terpin Hydrate Linctus Composition

THEORY

Terpin hydrate is an expectorant, commonly used to loosen mucus and ease congestion in patients presenting with acute or chronic bronchitis, and related pulmonary conditions. It is derived from sources such as turpentine, oregano, thyme, and eucalyptus.

Synonyms- Terpin monohydrate, Terpin (hydrate), p-Menthane-1,8-diol monohydrate

Terpin hydrate is highly soluble in water and hence alcohol is used to dissolve it.

Glycerine increases viscosity of linctus and is used as demulcent as it gives soothing effect.

Syrups is used as sweetening agent; **orange oil** is used as flavouring agent.

Terpin hydrate is sensitive to light and hence it should be packed in amber colour narrow mouth container.

TERPIN HYDRATE ELIXIR

FORMULA- Terpin hydrate (50gm), orange oil (0.2ml), glycerine (400ml), alcohol (425ml), syrup (100ml), purified water (q.s. or 1000ml)

MFD BY-

VG PHARMA

320, SOLAN INDUSTRIAL AREA, HIMACHAL PRADESH, INDIA

B. NO.- ZPM842X

MFG.D- 28/09/2022

EXP.D- 29/09/2022

MRP- Rs.50

INCL. ALL TAXES

STORAGE- Store in a well-closed container in a cool, dry place

Terpin Hydrate Linctus Sample Label

PROCEDURE

1. Terpin Hydrate was dissolved in a mixture of alcohol and Glycerine.
2. Then orange oil syrup was added, and volume made up with purified water.
3. The elixir was passed through a muslin cloth to obtain a clear solution.

CATEGORY

Expectorant

DOSE

As directed by physician.

USES

- Chronic bronchitis
- Pneumonia
- Chronic obstructive pulmonary disease
- Formulated with anti- tussive as combined preparation

STORAGE

Store in a well-closed container in a cool, dry place.

RESULT

Terpin hydrate linctus was prepared and dispensed.

VIVA- QUESTIONS

1. ***What is linctus?***
2. ***What is the most commonly used vehicle for preparation of linctus?***
3. ***What is use of terpin hydrate?***
4. ***What is synonym for terpin hydrate linctus?***
5. ***What is chemical formula for terpin hydrate?***

CHAPTER SEVEN

EXPERIMENT 7

AIM - To Prepare and dispense Iodine Throat Paint (Mandl's Paint).

MATERIAL REQUIREMENTS - Weighing balance, beaker, stirrer, glass mortar and pestle, measuring cylinder, potassium iodide, iodine, water, alcohol, peppermint oil, glycerine etc.

FORMULA

INGREDIENTS	QUANTITY USED	ROLE OF INGREDIENTS
Terpin hydrate	50gm	Expectorant
Orange oil	0.2ml	Flavouring agent
Glycerine	400ml	Demulcent
Alcohol	425ml	Solublizer
Syrup	100ml	Sweetening agent
Purified water	q.s. or 1000ml	Vehicle

Iodine Throat Paint (Mandl's Paint) Composition

THEORY

Throat paints are viscous solutions and dispersions, or one or more active ingredients intended for application to the mucosa of the throat or mouth. Iodine throat paint is also called as "Painting the External Throat" with iodine can reduce pain of the throat, may curb, and even eliminate throat infections, boosts overall immune functions, and help with conditions such as tonsilitis, pharyngitis, laryngitis and more. Iodine is a naturally occurring mineral that the body needs to produce hormones and control body's metabolism. In a liquid form, it is also used as an antibacterial agent and anti- inflammatory.

Iodine is slightly soluble in water and hence potassium iodide is used. When potassium iodide reacts with iodine it forms polyiodides which are soluble in water and solution becomes monophasic. Reaction between iodine and potassium iodide takes place as follows:

I2 (Iodine) + K1(Potassium Iodide) I2KI (Potassium mono iodide)

2I2 (Iodine)+ + K1(Potassium Iodide) 2I2KI (Potassium di iodide)

3I2 (Iodine)+ + K1(Potassium Iodide) 3I2KI (Potassium di iodide)

Glycerine is commonly used because it increases viscosity of the preparation, and the preparation adheres well to the mucous membrane of mouth and throat. It also gives a sweet taste and warm sensation to the inflamed area. **Alcohol** is used as co- solvent and increases the solubility of iodine is water, it also helps in dissolution of peppermint oil in it.

TERPIN HYDRATE ELIXIR

FORMULA- Terpin hydrate (50gm), orange oil (0.2ml), glycerine (400ml), alcohol (425ml), syrup (100ml), purified water (q.s. or 1000ml)

MFD BY-

VG PHARMA

320, SOLAN INDUSTRIAL AREA,
HIMACHAL PRADESH, INDIA

B. NO.- ZPM842X

MFG.D- 28/09/2022

EXP.D- 29/09/2022

MRP- Rs.50

INCL. ALL TAXES

STORAGE- Store in a well-closed container in a cool, dry place

Iodine Throat Paint (Mandl's Paint) Sample Label

PROCEDURE

1. Weigh required quantity of iodine and transfer unto glass mortar and triturate to get fine powder.
2. Weigh and dissolve required quantity of potassium iodide in water.
3. To this solution, add fine powdered iodine with continuous stirring.
4. In another beaker containing alcohol, add requires quantity of peppermint oil and half the quantity of glycerine. Add this solution to above iodine and potassium iodide solution with continuous stirring.
5. Pour content into the measuring cylinder and make up volume up to 20ml by addition of glycerine.
6. Transfer the contents to amber coloured wide mouth bottle, close it tightly with plastic screw cap, label and submit.

CATEGORY

In the treatment of pharyngitis, laryngitis and follicular tonsilitis.

STORAGE

Store in tightly closed container in cool and dark place.

DIRECTION

Apply with the help of soft brush or cotton swab. Food and water before and after application of throat paint should be avoided for 1 hour.

RESULT

Iodine throat paint was prepared and dispensed.

VIVA- QUESTIONS

1. *What is synonym of iodine throat paint?*
2. *What is composition of Mandl's paint?*
3. *How is solubility of iodine enhanced in Mandl's paint?*
4. *Paints are for external or internal application?*
5. *What is use of glycerine in iodine throat paint?*

CHAPTER EIGHT

EXPERIMENT 8

AIM : To prepare and evaluate 30 ml of cresol with soap solution.

MATERIAL REQUIRED - Cresol, vegetable oil, potassium hydroxide (KOH), water, beaker, glass rod and measuring cylinders

FORMULA

INGREDIENTS	STANDARD FORMULA	WORKING FORMULA	ROLE OF INGREDIENTS
Cresol	50ml	15ml	Disinfectant
Vegetable oil	18ml	5.4ml	Source of fatty acid
Potassium hydroxide	4.2g	1.26g	Alkali for soap formation
Purified water q.s. to produce	100ml	30ml	Solvent/ vehicle

Cresol with soap solution composition

THEORY

Pharmaceutical solutions are defined as liquids containing one or more soluble chemical substances dissolved in purified water intended for internal or external use.

Cresol (m-cresol) also 3- methyl phenol is an organic compound that is used as a house disinfectant. It is a colourless, viscous liquid. It is obtained from coal tar or petroleum.

Saponification is the process of manufacturing soap by reaction of vegetable oil or animal fat with NaOH and KOH (a solution of alkali). A soap solution increases the solubility of cresol due to the micelles present in the soap. A solution of cresol and soap is known as Lysol.

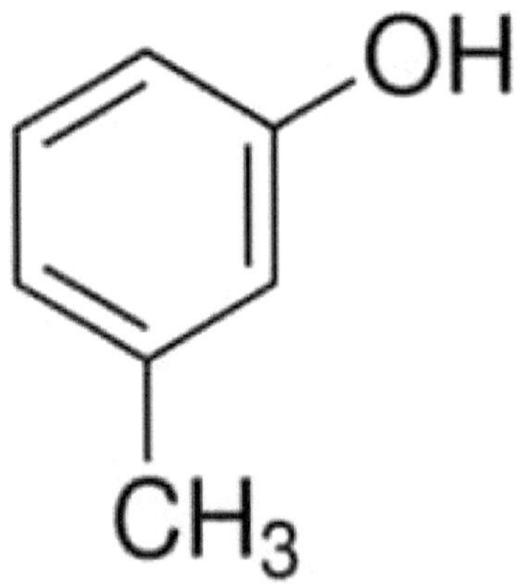

Structure of m-cresol

Structure of m-cresol

CRESOL SOAP SOLUTION IP 30ml

CRYSOL

DISINFECTANT

INGREDIENTS- CRESOL (15ml), VEGETABLE OIL (5.4ml), POTASSIUM HYDROXIDE (1.26gm), PURIFIRED WATER (30ml)

STORE PROTECTED FROM LIGHT

FOR EXTERNAL USE ONLY	KEEP OUT OF REACH OF CHILDREN

MFD BY- VG PHARMA, 320, SOLAN INDUSTRIAL AREA, HIMACHAL PRADESH, INDIA	**B. NO.**- A2MK6F
	MFG.D- 22/09/2022
	EXP.D- 22/09/2022
	MRP- Rs.43.00
REG NO- 1247892	INCL. ALL TAXES

Cresol with soap solution Sample Label

PROCEDURE-

1. Dissolve KOH in distilled water. Add vegetable oil in the solution and heat it over the water bath.
2. Heating is continued until the small part is dissolved in water without the separation of oil phase.

3. Add cresol to the above soap solution and mix thoroughly.
4. Add distilled water to produce 30ml.

CATEGORY

Disinfectant

PRECAUTIONS

- Not to be used near infants such as nursery, children ward etc.
- Not to be used in places where food is prepared and served.

DIRECTION

For external use only.

USE

Disinfectant

STORAGE

Protect from light, keep away from children.

RESULT

30 ml of Lysol was prepared and dispensed.

VIVA- QUESTIONS

1. ***What are solutions?***
2. ***What are advantages of solutions?***
3. ***What is cresol chemically?***
4. ***What are disinfectants?***
5. ***How much cresol is present in Lysol?***
6. ***What is role of vegetable oil in preparation for cresol with soap solution?***
7. ***What precautions are suggested while using cresol with soap solution?***

CHAPTER NINE

EXPERIMENT 9

AIM : To prepare and dispense 50 ml of strong ammonium acetate solution (CH3COONH4).

MATERIAL REQUIRED- Glacial acetic acid, ammonium bicarbonate, ammonium solution (strong), purified water, glass rod, measuring cylinder

THEORY

Ammonium acetate is also known as spirit of mindererus in aqueous solution. It is used in chemical analysis, textile dyeing and preserving meats. It is a diuretic (a drug that increases the volume of urine by promoting the excretion of salt and water from the kidney). It can also be used as diaphoretic (drug that causes increase in sweating) in febrile conditions such as influenza, acute pharyngitis etc. expectorants are medications or natural ingredients that help clear mucus from the airways. Eg strong ammonium acetate.

pH range of bromomethyl blue is 6.0 (yellow) to 7.6 (blue) and of bromothymol blue it is red below pH 1.2, yellow between pH 2.8 and 8.0 and blue above 9.6.

Glacial acetic acid reacts with ammonium bicarbonate and produce ammonium acetate:

CH3COOH (Glacial acetic acid) + NH4HCO3 (Ammonium bicarbonate) results in
CH3COONH4 (Ammonium acetate) + H2O+ CO2

INGREDIENTS	QUANTITY PRESCRIBED	QUANITITY USED	ROLE OF INGREDIENGT
Glacial acetic acid (CH3COOH)	453g	22.65g	Acid
Ammonium bicarbonate (NH4HCO3)	470g	23.5g	Alkali
Strong ammonium solution	100ml or q.s. to adjust pH	5ml or q.s. to adjust pH	Alkali
Bromothymol blue	1-2 drops	1-2 drops	Colouring agent
Thymol blue	1-2 drops	1-2 drops	Colouring agent
Distilled water	1000ml	50ml	Solvent

Ammonium acetate solution Composition

PROCEDURE

1. Dissolve ammonium bicarbonate in glacial acetic acid and water.
2. Strong ammonium solution is added to the above solution to adjust the pH to 7.4.
3. Resulting solution was withdrawn and to one drop of solution 10 drops of water was added.
4. In one beaker, bromothymol blue was added to give blue colour whereas to another thymol blue was added to give yellow colour.
5. To the prepared solution add distilled water to produce 50 ml.

STRONG AMMONIUM ACETATE IP 50 ml

AMONIUMATE

INGREDIENTS: GLACIAL ACETATIC ACID (22.65gm), AMMONIUM BICARBONATE (23.5gm), AMMONIUM SOLUTION (5ml max. or q.s.), PURIFIED WATER (50ml or q.s.)

STORAGE: STORE PROTECTED FROM LIGHT

USAGE: AS DIRECTED BY PHYSICIAN

MFD BY-

VG PHARMA

320, SOLAN INDUSTRIAL AREA, HIMACHAL PRADESH, INDIA

REG NO- 1247892

B. NO.- KG112V2403

MFG.D- 06/10/2020

EXP.D- 06/10/2022

MRP- Rs.199.00

INCL. ALL TAXES

Ammonium Acetate Solution Sample Label

CATEGORY

Diuretic, mild expectorant, and diaphoretic

DIRECTION

Take solution as directed by physician.

STORAGE

Protect from light in cool and dry place.

RESULT

50ml of strong ammonium acetate solution was prepared.

VIVA- QUESTIONS

1. *What is synonym of strong ammonium acetate solution?*
2. *What is strength of strong ammonium acetate solution?*
3. *What are uses of strong ammonium acetate solution?*
4. *Why are two alkalis used while preparation of strong ammonium acetate solution?*
5. *What are marketed formulations of solutions?*
6. *What are uses of strong ammonium acetate solution?*

CHAPTER TEN

EXPERIMENT 10

AIM : To prepare and dispense 50 ml of aqueous iodine solution (Lugol's solution).

MATERIAL REQUIRED- Iodine, potassium iodide (KI), water, beaker, glass rod and measuring cylinder

FORMULA

INGREDIENTS	QUANTITY PRESCRIBED	QUANTITY USED	ROL OF INGREDIENT
Potassium iodide (KI)	100gm	5gm	Solublizer
Iodine (I2)	50gm	2.5gm	Antiseptic
Distilled water	1000ml	50ml	Vehicle

Iodine solution (Lugol's solution) Composition

THEORY

Pharmaceutical solutions are defined as the liquids containing one or more soluble chemicals substance dissolved in purified water intended for internal or external use. Lugol's solution is an aqueous solution of iodine and KI. It is taken by mouth is used to treat thyrotoxicosis until surgery can be carried out, protect the thyroid gland from radioactivity of iodine and to treat iodine deficiency.

Iodine does not dissolve in water because water is extremely polar solution, while iodine exists in diatomic form (I2) and is therefore non- polar. Due to this reason, we add KI that forms polyhalide ion (I3—). KI forms a complex with I2 and helps it to get dissolved in water.

Lugol's solution may be given to treat goitre.

PROCEDURE

1. Dissolve potassium iodide (KI) in about 20-30 ml in distilled water.
2. Add iodine(I2) and heat gently with constant mixing until iodine is dissolved.
3. To the prepared solution add distilled water to procedure.

<table>
<tr><td colspan="2">

AQUEOUS IODINE SOLUTION IP 50ml

LUZOL

INGREDIENTS: POTASSIUM IODIDE (5gm), IODINE (2.5gm), PURIFIED WATER (50ml or q.s.)

STORAGE: STORE PROTECTED FROM LIGHT IN ORIGINAL CONTAINER

DIRECTION: AS DIRECTED BY PHYSICIAN

</td></tr>
<tr><td>

MFD BY-

VG PHARMA

320, SOLAN INDUSTRIAL AREA, HIMACHAL PRADESH, INDIA

REG NO- 1247892

</td><td>

B. NO.- KG3122VL

MFG.D- 06/10/2020

EXP.D- 06/10/2022

MRP- Rs.117.49

INCL. ALL TAXES

</td></tr>
</table>

Iodine solution (Lugol's solution) Sample Label

CATEGORY

For internal use in the treatment of simple goitre, for external use as an antiseptic.

USE

Source of iodine

STORAGE

Protect from light

RESULT

50 ml of aqueous iodine solution was prepared and dispensed.

VIVA- QUESTIONS

1. *What is synonym of aqueous iodine solution?*
2. *What are the uses of aqueous iodine solution*
3. *Why is aqueous iodine solution stored in amber glass bottle?*
4. *Why is potassium iodide used in Lugol's solution?*
5. *What are pharmaceutical solutions?*
6. *What are the uses of aqueous iodine solution?*

CHAPTER ELEVEN

EXPERIMENT 11

AIM - To prepare and supply 50ml of calamine lotion IP1966.

APPARATUS REQUIRED

Mortar pestle, beaker, stirrer, measuring cylinder

CHEMICALS REQUIRED

Calamine, bentonite, liquified phenol, ferrous oxide, zinc oxide, sodium citrate, glycerine, rose water

THEORY

Calamine is basically ZnCO3 mixed with suitable quantity of ferrous oxide (Fe2O3) to impart pink colour.

Zinc oxide (ZnO) has mild astringent, protectant, and antiseptic action. It is widely used in dusting powder, lotions and ointments made for treatment of skin diseases such as eczema, ringworm, psoriasis.

Bentonite is native colloidal hydrated aluminium silicate; it swells and imparts viscosity.

Sodium citrate is added to the preparation prevent the preparation from being viscous.

Liquified phenol is mild antiseptic.

Glycerine act as hygroscopic and humectant agent.

SNo.	INGREDIENTS	QUANITY USED
1.	Calamine	150g
2.	Bentonite	30g
3.	Liquid phenol	5ml
4.	Sodium citrate	5ml
5.	Zinc oxide (ZnO)	50gm
6.	Glycerine	50ml
7.	Rose water	q.s. to 1000ml

Calamine Lotion IP1966 Composition

PROCEDURE

1. Mix the weighed quantity of calamine, zinc oxide and bentonite in a mortar.
2. Triturate it with solution of sodium citrate in about 700ml of rose water.
3. Add the required quantity of liquified phenol and glycerine and mix well.
4. To this add more vehicle to produce required volume roughly so as to get uniform preparation.

CALAMINE LOTION IP 1966	
IP FORMULA: Calamine (7.5g), bentonite (1.5g), liquid paraffin (0.25ml), ZnO (2.5 gm), sodium citrate (2.5g), glycerine (2.5g), rose water (50ml) **STORAGE:** Store in well closed container.	**MFG Date**- 18/08/17 **EXP Date**- 17/ 08/18 **Batch No**- 999 **MFG By**- PM Pharmaceutical Pvt Ltd. **MFG License**- 909 **MRP**- Rs. 100 **DIRECTION- SHAKE WELL BEFORE USE**

Calamine Lotion IP1966 Sample Label

CALCULATIONS

1. **Calamine**- 150/1000×50= 7.5g
2. **Bentonite**- 30/1000×50= 1.5g
3. **Liquid phenol**- 5/1000×50= 0.25g
4. **Zinc oxide**- 50/1000×50= 2.5g
5. **Glycerine**- 50/1000×50= 2.5ml
6. **Rose water**- 1000/1000×50= 50ml

STORAGE

Store it in well closed container.

CATEGORY

Astringent and protective

DIRECTION

Apply to affected part without rubbing whenever necessary.

USES

This lotion is used as an astringent. It acts as smoothening agent and gives relief during pain and itching during skin irritates. It is also used in ringworm infection and eczema.

RESULT

50 ml of calamine lotion IP1966 was prepared and labelled.

PRECAUTIONS

1. Apparatus used should be washed and dried.
2. Chemicals should be weighed properly and accurately.

VIVA- QUESTIONS

1. ***Define suspensions.***

2. ***What are advantages and disadvantages of suspensions.***
3. ***What is difference between calamine lotion I.P. and calamine lotion B.P.?***
4. ***What do you mean by astringent?***
5. ***What are the precautions taken while use of calamine lotion?***
6. ***How is calamine lotion applied to body?***

CHAPTER TWELVE

EXPERIMENT 12

AIM : To prepare and supply magnesium hydroxide (MgOH) oral suspension (60ml).

APPARATUS - Mortar and pestle, stirrer, measuring cylinder, beaker

SYNONYM - Milk of magnesia, cream of magnesia, magnesium hydroxide

FORMULA

Light MgOH- 6ml

Distilled water- 60ml

THEORY

Mg (OH)2 is inorganic compound. It occurs in nature as mineral brucite. It is a white solid. It is common component of antacid such as milk of magnesia as well as laxative. It is used to treat symptoms like heart burn, upset stomach and indigestion. It may cause allergic reactions like swelling of face, lips. Tongue, difficulty in breathing etc.

Preparation of magnesium hydroxide by precipitation:

$MgSO_4 + 2NaOH$------ $Mg(OH)_2 + Na_2SO_4$

USES-

1. It is used an antacid and as a laxative.
2. Acne and oily skin can be treated.
3. It treats wounds, skin rashes, indigestion etc.
4. It is used as antidepressant.

PROCEDURE

In a pestle and mortar add MgO and 20ml water, triturate till a cream is formed. Add more water to make the volume.

<table>
<tr><th colspan="2">MAGNESIUM HYDROXIDE ORAL SUSPENSION</th></tr>
<tr><td>FORMULA- Light MgO (6g),
distilled water (q.s, or 60 ml)
CATEGORY- Antacid
USE- Used as an antacid and laxative
and as an antiperspirant.
STORAGE- Stored in well closed container
so as to prevent from moisture.</td><td>MFG Date- 22/09/17
EXP Date- 21/ 09/18
Batch No- 999
MFG By- MPH Pharmaceutical Pvt Ltd.
MFG License- ATTP999
MRP- Rs. 40
DIRECTION- SHAKE WELL BEFORE USE</td></tr>
</table>

Magnesium hydroxide (MgOH) oral suspension Sample Label

STORAGE

Stored so as to protect from moisture or at a temperature not exceeding 25˚C.

DIRECTION

Shake well before use.

RESULT

Mg (OH)2 oral suspension was prepared and labelled.

PRECAUTIONS

Weighing should be done accurately.

Apparatus should be dried and washed properly.

VIVA- QUESTIONS

1. ***What is the method of preparation of magnesium hydroxide by precipitation?***
2. ***What are the uses of magnesium hydroxide suspension?***
3. ***What are the general components of suspensions?***
4. ***What are the storage conditions for magnesium hydroxide suspension?***
5. ***What are the side effects of magnesium hydroxide?***

CHAPTER THIRTEEN

EXPERIMENT 13

AIM : To prepare and dispense Aluminium hydroxide gel.

APPARATUS AND CHEMICALS - Glass rod, stirrer, measuring cylinder, beaker, conical flask, burette, aluminium chloride

FORMULA

INGREDIENTS	QUANTITY GIVEN	QUANTITY USED	ACTIVITY
Aluminium Hydroxide	36gm	7.2g	Antacid
Sorbitol	7g	1.4g	Preservative
Methyl paraben	0.2g	0.04g	Preservative
Propyl paraben	0.2g	0.04g	Preservative
Saccharin	0.20g	0.04g	Sweetener
Peppermint oil	0.005ml	0.001ml	Flavouring agent
Alcohol	1ml	0.2ml	Solubilizer
Purified water	100ml	20ml	Vehicle

Aluminium hydroxide Gel composition

THEORY

Antacids are alkaline bases used to neutralize excess gastric Hcl associated with gastric and peptic ulcers. This, in turn, inactivates pepsin which functions optimally at low ph.

Aluminium hydroxide is an inorganic compound made up of aluminium ion and hydroxide ions. It is an amphoteric compound which means it can act as an acid as well as a base. Aluminium hydroxide minerals occur in nature. It holds the property of an antacid. The IUPAC name of the aluminium hydroxide is Aluminium trioxide.

Hydrophobicity is a property of aluminium hydroxide. In most cases, it produces lyophobic solutions. The hydrolysis of aluminium chloride can be used to prepare aluminium hydroxide gels.

$$3H_2O + AlCl_3 \text{ -------} Al(OH)_3 + 3HCl$$

Properties of Aluminium Hydroxide

- The Colour of aluminium hydroxide is white.
- Its density is 2.43 g/cm^3.
- Its melting point is 300 degrees Celsius.
- Its molar mass is 78.0036.

PROCEDURE

1. Prepare the 2% aluminium chloride solution (by adding 2g of aluminium chloride in 100 ml water).

2. Add 100 ml distilled water to the conical flask.
3. Boil the water with the help of the wire gauze.
4. Add 10 ml of the above prepared 2% aluminium chloride solution. Add this solution with the help of the dropper of the burette. As aluminium compounds are violent in nature.
5. Constantly stir the solution while adding aluminium chloride.
6. Heat the solution until you see a coloured solution. The colour of the aluminium hydroxide solution is white.
7. Leave the mixture for cooling at normal temperature.
8. The cooling solution is called aluminium hydroxide gel.
9. Precaution You Need to keep During Aluminium Hydroxide Gel Preparation
10. Clean the conical flask with a steaming process to avoid any kind of impurities.
11. The by-product (Hydrochloric Acid) formed in this reaction causes destabilization of the prepared gel. therefore, needs to be removed by the dialysis process.
12. Aluminium chloride solutions need to be added in a dropwise manner.

ALUMINIUM HYDROXIDE GEL

FORMULA- Aluminium Hydroxide (36gm), Preservatives, sweetener, Peppermint oil (0.005gm), distilled water (q.s. or 100 ml)	**MFG Date**- 22/09/17
	EXP Date- 21/ 09/18
CATEGORY- Antacid	**Batch No**- 999
USE- Used as an antacid and in stomach ulcers.	**MFG By**- MPH Pharmaceutical Pvt Ltd.
STORAGE- Stored in well closed container below 30 °c, avoid freezing	**MFG License**- ATTP999
	MRP- Rs. 100

Aluminium hydroxide Gel Sample Label

CATEGORY
Antacid
DOSE
7.5 to 15 ml
STORAGE
Store in the well-closed container below 30 °c, avoid freezing.

USES

- It is used for treating gastric ulcers.
- It serves as an intermediate compound in various reactions.
- It is used in the manufacturing of certain drugs.

RESULT
Aluminium hydroxide gel was prepared and dispensed.

VIVA- QUESTIONS

1. ***What are the types of solid suspensions?***
2. ***Enlist methods for evaluation of suspensions.***
3. ***What are the properties of aluminium hydroxide?***
4. ***What are antacids?***
5. ***What are the uses of aluminium hydroxide gel?***
6. ***What is the dose given for aluminium hydroxide gel?***

CHAPTER FOURTEEN

EXPERIMENT 14

AIM : To prepare and dispense 40 ml of turpentine emulsion.

THEORY

An emulsion is a colloid of two or more immiscible liquids where one liquid is called dispersed phase and other is called as dispersion medium. There are two basic types of emulsions-

1. ***Oil in water type:*** Where water is DM and oil is DP e.g., Milk, ice cream etc.
2. ***Water in oil type:*** Where water is DP and oil is DM. Eg butter, cold cream

Sometimes we add emulsifiers or emulsifying agents to stabilize the emulsions. An emulsifying agent is a compound or substance that acts as an interface between immiscible and forms stable emulsions. Common examples of emulsifying agents are albumin, soaps, egg yolk, gums, benzalkonium chloride, sodium docusate, glyceryl esters, detergents. Based on the size of droplets emulsions can be divided into 3 types-

1. Macroemulsions (0.1μm- 5μm)
2. Microemulsions (5μm)
3. Nanoemulsions

There are 2 main types of method of preparation of emulsions:

1. Wet gum method- The proportion of oil, water and emulsifiers are 4:2:1. In this method, 1 part is triturated with 2 parts of water to form a mucilage, then 4 parts of oil are added slowly in portions while triturating. After all the oil is added, the mixture is triturated for several minutes to form primary emulsions.
2. Dry gum method- The proportion of oil, water and emulsifiers are 4:2:1. In a mortar, 1 part gum is levigated with 4 parts of oil until the powder is thoroughly wetted, then 2 parts of water are added all the once and mixture is triturated until the primary emulsion is formed creamy white and produces a crackling sound as it is triturated.Using a mortar and pestle the thick and primary emulsion is made first in the ratio of oil, water and gum as follows:

	OIL	WATER	GUM
Fixed oil	4	2	1 eg- almond, castor oil etc
Mineral oil	3	2	1 eg- liquid paraffin
Volatile oil	2	2	1 eg- turpentine, peppermint, and cinnamon

Turpentine Emulsion

Several factors are considered

We need to specify:

1. Whether it is o/w or w/o emulsion.
2. Use of the product i.e., whether it is for external or internal or injectable use.

CONSIDER

1. Ingredients taking into accounting the chemical structure, physical properties (melting point, solubility, and stability).
2. Dose of preparation (which has an impact on overall volume).
3. Incompatibilities of ingredients.
4. Choice of emulgents.

PROCEDURE

1. Make sure that the glassware is dry.
2. **Preparation of primary emulsion-** Take oil and powdered gum acacia in a dried mortar and pestle and mix the gum with the help of pestle.
3. Add purified water drop wise with continuous trituration in only one direction.
4. After clicking sound primary emulsion is prepared.
5. Now secondary emulsion is prepared by slowly incorporating distilled water to produce 50ml.

TURPENTINE EMULSION IP 40ml, 20% V/V

TURPENT EMULS

INGREDIENTS: TURPENTINE OIL (8ml), GUM ACACIA (8gm), PURIFIED WATER (50ml or q.s.)

STORAGE: STORE PROTECTED FROM LIGHT IN ORIGINAL CONTAINER

USAGE: AS DIRECTED BY PHYSICIAN

MFD BY-
VG PHARMA
320, SOLAN INDUSTRIAL AREA, HIMACHAL PRADESH, INDIA
REG NO- 1247892

B. NO.- 1789EGQ7
MFG.D- 13/10/2020
EXP.D- 13/10/2022
MRP- Rs.201.42

FOR EXTERNAL USE ONLY

NOT TO BE APPLIED ON BROKEN SKIN
"SHAKE WELL BEFORE USE"

Turpentine Emulsion Sample Label

CALCULATIONS

INGREDIENTS	QUANTITY PRESCRIBED	QUANTITY USED	ROLE OF INGREDIENTS
Turpentine oil	20ml	8g	Counter irritant and rubefacient
Gum acacia	10g	4g	Stabilizer
Purified water	100ml	40ml	Vehicle

Turpentine Emulsion Composition

CATEGORY

Counter- irritant and rubefacient.

USE

Carminative

STORAGE

Store in well closed container, protect from sunlight.

CONTAINS

20%v/v turpentine oil

RESULT

40ml of turpentine was prepared and dispensed.

VIVA- QUESTIONS

1. ***Define emulsions. What are the advantages and disadvantages of emulsions?***
2. ***What is the use of gum acacia in turpentine emulsion?***
3. ***What are the types of emulsions?***
4. ***What are the two main method of preparation for emulsions?***
5. ***What is the use of turpentine emulsion?***
6. ***What are the storage conditions for turpentine emulsion?***

CHAPTER FIFTEEN

EXPERIMENT 15

AIM : To Prepare Liquid Paraffin Emulsion by Wet Gum Method.

APPARATUS REQUIRED- Mortar and pestle, stirrer, measuring cylinder, beaker

FORMULA

Liquid paraffin- 30ml

Water- 100ml or q.s.

OIL	WATER	GUM
4	2	1
30	15	7.5

Liquid Paraffin Emulsion Composition

THEORY

Liquid paraffin is a type of medicine called a laxative. It works by lubricating and softening the stools. This helps stools to move out slowly through the bowel. Liquid paraffin is considered to have limited usefulness as an occasional laxative but it not suitable for daily use as it can seep from anus and can cause irritation.

Liquid paraffin acts as a laxative.

Gum acacia acts as an emulsifying agent.

PROCEDURE

Wet Gum Method:

1. Thoroughly clean and dry mortar and pestle.
2. Weigh out 8g of acacia and transfer it to mortar.
3. Add 10ml of water and triturate it.
4. Then add 30ml of liquid paraffin in small quantity at a time and triturate it after each addition.
5. Triturate briskly without stopping and without changing the direction until a clicking sound is produced and product becomes white or nearly white. This is called primary emulsion.
6. Add remaining quantity of water with constant trituration so as to get homogeneous product.

<table>
<tr><th colspan="2">LIQUID PARAFFIN EMULSION</th></tr>
<tr><td>IP FORMULA- Liquid paraffin (30ml),
gum acacia (8g),
water q.s, or 100ml)
CATEGORY- Laxative
DOSE- Aa prescribed by physician
STORAGE- Store below 25°C and do not refrigerate.</td><td>MFG Date- 08/09/17
EXP Date- 07/ 09/18
Batch No- 999
MFG By- MP Pharmaceutical Pvt Ltd.
MFG License- 999
MRP- Rs. 40
DIRECTION- SHAKE WELL BEFORE USE</td></tr>
</table>

Liquid Paraffin Emulsion Sample Label

CATEGORY

Laxative

DIRECTION

Shake well before use

STORAGE

Store below 25°C and do not refrigerate.

RESULT

Liquid paraffin was prepared and supplied.

PRECAUTIONS

1. Apparatus used should be properly washed and dried.
2. Chemicals we use should be weighed and measured accurately.

VIVA- QUESTIONS

1. *What are the uses liquid paraffin?*
2. *Define laxatives.*
3. *What is difference between liniment and lotion?*
4. *What are the storage conditions for liquid paraffin emulsion?*
5. *What is the method of preparation for liquid paraffin emulsion?*
6. *Why is liquid paraffin passed through homogenizer?*

CHAPTER SIXTEEN

EXPERIMENT 16

AIM : To prepare and dispense Oral rehydration salts (ORS) according to WHO formula.

MATERIAL REQUIRED- Sodium chloride (NaCl) powder, potassium chloride (Kcl) powder, sodium citrate dihydrate, pestle mortar.

THEORY-

Oral rehydration solution (ORS) is used to treat dehydration caused by diarrhoea a common illness in travellers.

Diarrhoea is the disorder causes us to pass more stools than usual or excessive vomiting. Diarrhoea is caused due to dehydration when a person's body losses fluid which contains salts like Na, K etc. Na is both an electrolyte and mineral. It helps to keep water and electrolyte balance in the body. It is also important for proper functioning of nerves and muscles. About 85% of Na is found in blood and lymph. A hormone secreted by adrenal gland; aldosterone regulates the kidney for maintaining Na level in the body. K is also important electrolyte for normal functioning of cells, regulating heartbeat, ensuring proper functioning of nerves and muscles, vitals for synthesizing of carbohydrate and proteins.

Another important chemical released during diarrhoea is citrate ion. We add sodium citrate into ORS which dissociated into Na+ and citrate anions, which are metabolised to bicarbonate ions, resulting in increased concentration of bicarbonate in plasma. In addition, it may also increase blood volume, facilitating anti- urolithic effect.

Chloride too gets deficient in diarrhoea. It is one of the most important electrolytes, it helps in maintaining fluid balance inside and outside of cells, proper blood volume, blood pressure and ph of body fluids.

During diarrhoea, the glucose level of the body decreases. Glucose is the main source of energy for our body. Every cell of the body requires adequate amount of glucose to perform their respective function. Excess glucose is stored in little bundles called glycogen in the liver and muscles.

Normal limits of:

1. Sodium- normal blood sodium level is 135-145Meg/l.
2. Potassium- normal blood potassium level is 3.6- 5.2 mml/l.
3. Citrate ions- 0.05- 0.3 mM.
4. Glucose- normal blood sugar level ranges from 4.8- 5.4 mml/l and fasting upto 7.8 mmol/l 2 hours after eating.

ORAL REHYDRATION SOLUTION, 50gm

ENERGILE

INGREDIENTS: SODIUM CHLORIDE (6.3g), POTASSIUM CHLORIDE (3.7g), SODIUM CITRATE DIHYDRATE (7.0g), GLUCOSE (33.0g)

STORAGE: STORE IN DRY PLACE, NOT ABOVE 30°C

MFD BY-

VG PHARMA

320, SOLAN INDUSTRIAL AREA, HIMACHAL PRADESH, INDIA

REG NO- 1247892

B. NO.- KVG26954

MFG.D- 17/10/2020

EXP.D- 17/10/2022

MRP- Rs.21.70

INCL. ALL TAXES

Oral rehydration salts (ORS) Sample Label

PROCEDURE-

1. Weigh each ingredient on individual butter paper suing class 2 dispensing balance.
2. Transfer NaCl, Kcl and sodium citrate ingredients starting with the lowest weight to the porcelain mortar.
3. Mix with pestle and approximately equal quantity of glucose was added and mixed again and at lost add remaining quantity of glucose.
4. Pack the resulting powder blend in a moisture resistant paper (butter paper).
5. Label it completely.

S No.	INGREDIENTS	WEIGHT PRESRIBED	RELATIVE MOLECULAR MASS	WEIGHT TAKEN (gm)
1.	NaCl	2.6g/l	58.44	6.3
2.	KCl	1.5g/l	74.55	3.7
3.	Sodium citrate ($C6H5Na3O7.2H2O$)	2.9g/l	294.10	7.0
4.	Glucose, anhydrous	13.5g/l	180.20	33.0
	Total	20.5		50

Oral rehydration salts (ORS) Composition

RESULT

50gm of ORS was prepared and dispensed.

VIVA- QUESTIONS

1. ***What is ORS?***
2. ***What is diarrhoea?***
3. ***Define cathartic.***
4. ***What do you mean by oral rehydration therapy?***
5. ***What are the normal limits and role of sodium and potassium in body?***

CHAPTER SEVENTEEN

EXPERIMENT 17

AIM-To prepare and submit 100g of effervescent granules.

APPARATUS REQUIRED- Mortar and pestle, China dish, sieve of sieve no 40 and 6.

FORMULA-

Sodium phosphate dried and powdered- 200g

Sodium bicarbonate in dry powder- 477g

Tartaric acid in dry powder- 252g

Citric acid mono hydrate- 162g

THEORY-

Eno is an antacid which contains a mixture of sodium bicarbonate (NaHCO3), citric acid, sodium carbonate. Upon addition of water, the citric acid will start to dissociate and eventually becomes reactive. It can convert bicarbonates into CO2 and water. It is very handy after those spicy dinners after which you feel the need to calm your stomach acid. It reduces the stomach bloating and burning sensation in oesophagus.

Sodium phosphate is used as cathartic and other ingredients forms effervescent in water.

PROCEDURE-

1. Powder citric acid and mix well with dried sodium phosphate and tartaric acid.
2. Add sodium bicarbonate to above mixture and heat gently.
3. Transfer and heat the mixture in china dish gently.
4. Stir well it gets damp.
5. Press damp mass through sieve no 6.
6. Dry granules at a temperature not exceeding 54˚C.
7. Pass the dry granules through sieve no 40.
8. Pack dried uniform size granules in a wide mouth bottle and label.

EFFERVESCENT GRANULES	
FORMULA- Sodium phosphate (20g), sodium bicarbonate (47.7g), tartaric acid (25.2g), citric acid monohydrate (16.2g)	**MFG Date**- 20/10/17 **EXP Date**- 19/ 10/18 **Batch No**- A1P99
USES- Antacid, also called as Eno fruit salt and gas go and used in constipation.	**MFG By**- PM Pharmaceutical Pvt Ltd. **MFG License**- 99849 **MRP**- Rs. 6

Enter Caption

CALCULATIONS-
Sodium phosphate- 200/1000×100= 20g
Sodium bicarbonate- 477/1000×100= 47.7g
Tartaric acid- 252/1000×100= 25.2g
Citric acid monohydrate- 162/1000×100= 16.2g
CATEGORY-
Antacid
USES-
For acidity
DIRECTION-
Shake well before use and mix with water and consume simultaneously.
RESULT- Effervescent granules (100g) was prepared and supplied.
VIVA- QUESTIONS

1. ***What are effervescent granules?***
2. ***What is composition of effervescent granules?***
3. ***What are the uses of effervescent granules?***
4. ***What is direction for use of effervescent granules?***
5. ***What is use of sodium phosphate in effervescent granules?***

CHAPTER EIGHTEEN

EXPERIMENT 18

AIM- To prepare and label dusting powder/ talcum I.P.
APPARATUS REQUIRED- Mortar and pestle, sieve (of sieve size 80).
CHEMICAL REQUIRED: Purified talc, starch, zinc oxide, salicylic acid.
IP FORMULA

INGRIDIENTS	QUANTITY USED	ROLE OF INGREDIENT
Purified talc	50g	Absorbs moisture
Starch	25g	Absorbance and covering
Zinc Oxide	5g	Astringent
Salicylic acid	20g	Antiseptic

Composition of Dusting powder/ talcum

THEORY

Dusting powders are formulations which are intended to be applied on skin or on wounds especially for alloying irritation or absorbing moisture ingredients used in dusting powders are:

PURIFIED TALC - Talc absorbs moisture, oil and help in skin feel soft, fresh, cool, and dry. It helps to reduce friction and chafing that can irritate skin.

ZINC OXIDE - Zinc oxide is used as it has astringent and antiseptic properties and acts a skin protectant as it screens UVA and UVB.

SALICYLIC ACID - Salicylic acid is a powerful antiseptic and exert a strong inhibitory influence upon growth of micro-organism

STARCH - Starch is used as base for dusting powders and have absorbent properties.

PROCEDURE

1. Weigh the required quantity of starch, talc, zinc oxide and salicylic acid.
2. Mix them with in ascending weight order of weight.
3. Pass the mixed powder through sieve no. 80.
4. After sieving mix the contents again appropriate label and submit.

DUSTING POWDER

IP Formula: Purified talc (12.5g), Starch (6.25g), zinc oxide (125g), Salicylic acid (5g).

Uses: keep skin fresh, absorb oil and moisture, and treat various fungal infection like ringworm.

Storage: store it in well closed container.

Direction for use: apply product liberally

as often as necessary.

Warning – for external use only. Avoid

Mfg. Date- 25 Aug 2017

Exp. Date- 24 Aug 2018

Mfg. by- M.P Pharmaceutic Pvt. Ltd.

Batch No- 111AP47

MRP- ₹50/-

Dusting Powder/ Talcum powder Label

USES- Dusting powders are applied to body to help and moisture and to impart fragrance. These are also treated athlete's foot, jock, itch, ringworm etc.

STORAGE- Preserve in well closed container and it may be preserved in sealed paper.

CALCULATIONS-

To prepare 25g dusting powder-

1. Purified talc- 50/100 × 25= 12.5g
2. Starch- 25/100 × 25= 6.25g
3. Zin oxide- 5/100× 25= 1.25g
4. Salicylic acid- 20/100×25= 5

RESULT- Dusting powder was prepared and labelled.

PRECAUTIONS-

1. Apparatus used should be properly washed, cleaned, and dried.
2. Chemicals should be weighed accurately.

VIVA- QUESTIONS

1. ***What is dusting powder?***
2. ***Why is dusting powder passed through 80 mesh sieves?***
3. ***What is use of salicylic acid in dusting powder?***

4. ***What are the precautions taken while using dusting powder?***
5. ***What is the role of zinc oxide in dusting powder?***

CHAPTER NINETEEN

EXPERIMENT 19

AIM-To prepare and submit divided powder.

REQUIREMENTS- Aspirin, paracetamol, beaker, measuring cylinder, stirrer etc.

THEORY

Divided powder is divided into the prescribed number of doses and is given orally. Each dose (0.1–1.0 g) should be transferred to a powder paper. These are unit dose powders normally packed properly. Divided powder is more accurate dosage form than bulk powder because patient is not involved in measurement of dosage form.

Divided powders are commercially available in foil, cellophane, or paper packs.

FORMULA

INGREDIENTS	STANDARD FORMULA
Aspirin	300 mg
Paracetamol	150 mg

Composition of Divided Powder

PROCEDURE

1. Weigh the calculated number of aspirin and paracetamol.
2. Mix them thoroughly.
3. Weigh 450 mg of mixed powder.
4. Divide the powder into four equal parts.
5. Wrap in suitable size powder.

Rx

DIVIDED POWDER (20 ml)

FORMULA-

Aspirin 300 mg, Paracetamol 150 mg.

USES- keep skin fresh,

Absorb oil and moisture, and treat

various fungal infection like

Ringworm.

STORAGE- store it in well closed

MFG Date- 30 Aug 2020

EXP Date- 24 Aug 2022

Mfg. by- M.P Pharmaceutic Pvt. Ltd.

BATCH NO- 111BP49

MRP- ₹75/-

Direction for use: Apply product liberally

WARNING! – for external use only. Avoid contact with eyes

Divided powder Label

USES

Antacid, bulk laxative

STORAGE

Store in a well-closed container and keep in a cool place.

DIRECTION

Take one packet as directed by physician.

RESULT

Divided powder was prepared.

VIVA- QUESTIONS

1. ***What is divided powder?***
2. ***What is the use of aspirin in divided powder?***
3. ***How are divided powder available commercially?***
4. ***What is method of preparation for divided powder?***
5. ***What are the uses of divided powder?***
6. ***What is the storage condition for divided powder?***

CHAPTER TWENTY

EXPERIMENT 20

AIM - To prepare & dispense 10 glycero gelation suppositories of 1 gm each.
MATERIAL REQUIRED- Gelatine, glycerol, China dish, beaker, glass rod & measuring cylinder.
FORMULA

INGREDIENTS	QUANTITY GIVEN	QUANTITY TAKEN	ROLE OF INGREDIENT
Glycerine	70 g	0.7g	Laxative
Gelatine	16g	0.16g	Stiffness
Purified water Q.S.	1000g	10g	vehicle

Composition of Glycero Gelation Suppositories

THEORY

- Suppositories are solid dosage forms intended for insertion into body orifices where they melt, soften, or dissolve & exert localised or systemic effects.
- A suppository is a drug delivery system that is inserted into the rectum (rectal suppository), vagina (vaginal suppository) or urethra (urethral suppository), where it dissolves or melts.
- They are used to deliver both systematically of locally acting medications.
- The general principle is that the suppository is inserted as a solid, which melts or dissolves inside the body to deliver the medicine received by the many blood vessels that follow the large intestine.
- Laxatives, purgatives, or aperients are substances that loosen stools & increase bowel movements. They are used to treat & prevent constipation.
- Laxatives promote the elimination of soft, formed faeces whereas purgatives produce a more fluid evacuation. Eg: methylcellulose, psyllium, polycarbophil.

PROCEDURE

1. Clean the mould with soap & water.
2. Dry the mould & lubricate the mould with light mineral oil.
3. Heat the glycerine at a temperature of 100°c in a China dish.
4. Soak the gelatine in water for 5-10 minutes & then add the hot glycerine to the soaked gelatine.
5. Stir the mixture on a water bath for 15 mins or till a solution is obtained.
6. Remove from heat of allow the mixture to cool before pouring into the mould.

7. Overfill the cavities in the mould, cool at room temperature for 30 mins & then place in a refrigerator for 15-20 mins if the suppositories have not completely congealed.
8. Carefully remove excess with a hot spatula or knife. Remove suppositories from mould.
9. Using only perfect specimens, weigh the suppositories & record the total weight. Calculate the average suppository weight.

10 GLYCERO GELTIN SUPPOSITORIES

INGREDIENTS- Glycerine (0.7g), gelatine (0.16g), purified water q.s. (10g),

DIRECTION- LUBRICATE WITH WATER & INSERT THROUGH RECTUM AT BEDTIME.

FOR RECTAL USE ONLY

MFG BY- KV PHARMA
320, SOLAN INDUSTRIAL AREA,
HIMACHAL PRADESH, INDIA
REG. NO.- 1247984

BATCH NO- 111AP47
MFG Date- 27/10/2020
EXP Date- 27/10/2023
MRP- ₹75.69/-

Glycero Gelation Suppositories Label

DIRECTION

For rectal use only. Lubricate with water of insert through rectum at bedtime.

USE

Laxative

STORAGE

Store in a cool place.

RESULT

10 glycero gelatine suppositories were prepared of dispensed with a weight of 1g each.

VIVA- QUESTIONS

1. *Define suppositories. Give its types.*
2. *What are advantages and disadvantaged of suppositories?*
3. *What are different components of suppositories?*
4. *What is composition of glycero gelation suppositories?*
5. *What are storage conditions for glycero gelation suppositories?*

CHAPTER TWENTY-ONE

EXPERIMENT 21

AIM- To preparation and evaluation of Zinc Oxide suppository using Coca butter as a suppository base.
MATERIAL REQUIRED-Evaporating dish, glass rod, Suppository mould, Zinc Oxide, cocoa butter etc.
FORMULA

INGREDIENTS	QUANTITY GIVEN	ACTIVITY
Zinc Oxide	120 mg	Astringent
Cocoa butter	q.s to	Suppository base

Enter Caption

PROCEDURE

1. The mould was lubricated with soft soap and kept in an inverted position for some time.
2. The quantity of base required was calculated by taking into consideration the displacement value of Zinc oxide and the capacity of mould. zinc oxide was passed through a sieve 60 mesh
3. Theobroma oil was melted in an evaporating dish on a warm water bath at a temperature not exceeding 36˚C. Zinc oxide was added to the molten cocoa butter and mixed.
4. The mixture was poured into the pre-lubricated mould and allowed to set on an ice bath for 5 minutes. the Excess was Scrap off. Suppositories were removed and packed in boxes lined by means of a separator.

Rx

ZINC OXIDE SUPPOSITORY USING COCA BUTTER

FORMULA-

Zinc oxide 120 mg, Coca butter as per q.s

STORAGE- Store in a cool and dry place

MFD BY-

VG PHARMA

320, SOLAN INDUSTRIAL AREA, HIMACHAL PRADESH, INDIA

REG NO- 1247892

B. NO.- KG112V2403

MFG.D- 03/10/2020

EXP.D- 09/10/2022

MRP- Rs.199.00

INCL. ALL TAXES

For rectal use only. Use 1 at night and 1 in the morning after defecation. Insert suppository as high as possible in the rectum.

Enter Caption

PRECAUTION

Invert lubricated mould for some time before filling.

CATEGORY

Astringent or Laxative

CONTAINER / STORAGE

Store in a cool and dry place.

LABELLINGDIRECTIONS

For rectal use only. Use 1 at night and 1 in the morning after defecation. Insert suppository as high as possible in the rectum.

RESULT

Zinc Oxide suppository using Coca butter as a suppository base was prepared.

VIVA- QUESTIONS

1. *Define suppositories. Give its types.*
2. *What are advantages and disadvantages of suppositories?*
3. *What is use of zinc oxide suppository?*
4. *What is use of zinc oxide suppository?*
5. *What are applications of suppositories*
6. *What are different quality control test for suppositories?*

CHAPTER TWENTY-TWO

EXPERIMENT 22

AIM- To prepare sulphur ointment (10g).

REQUIREMENT- Ointment slab, ointment spatula, precipitated sulphur, and simple ointment.

FORMULA

Precipitated Sulphur - 10g

Simple ointment - 90g

THEORY-

Ointment are homogeneous, semi- solid preparations intended for external application to the skin or mucous membrane. They are used as emollient or for the application of active ingredient to the skin for protective, therapeutic, or prophylactic purposes.

Sulphur ointment is used for several conditions and is used in formulations mainly used for scabies and seborrheic dermatitis. It may kill adult scabies mites. It is used only when permethrin or other medicines cannot be used. It is used as it is thought to be very much safe, but it may day the skin. In this preparation sulphur ointment is used as absorption base. As precipitated sulphur is hydrophobic in nature, it is insoluble in simple ointment which is hydrophilic in nature. Hence, sulphur ointment is prepared by levigation on ointment slab or triturated in dry mortar.

PROCEDURE- Triturate the precipitated sulphur with small amount of simple ointment on an ointment slab. Gradually add the remainder of simple ointment until a homogenous mass is obtained.

SULPHUR OINTMENT (10g)

FORMULA- Precipitated Sulphur (1g), Simple ointment (9g)

USES- Fungicidal, used in treatment of scabies and ringworm infection and treat

MFG Date-25Aug2017

EXP Date- 24 Aug 2018

MFG by- MPH Pharma company Pvt. Ltd.

BATCH NO- AIP 419

MFG. LICENSE NO- ZA4P

MRP- ₹85/-

Sulphur ointment Label

CALCULATIONS

Since, we have to make only 10g of sulphur ointment, quality of medicaments used are-

Precipitated Sulphur: 10g×10/100 = 10g

Simple Ointment: 90g×10/100 = 9g

CATEGORY

In treatment of scabies and acne.

STORAGE

Store in cool and dry place.

DIRECTION

Apply on affected area as directed by physician.

USES

- Used as fungicidal
- Used in treatment of scabies.
- Used in treatment of ringworm infection.

RESULT

Sulphur ointment was prepared and supplied.

PRECAUTIONS

1. Mixing of sulphur and simple ointment.
2. Should be done carefully and completely so as to make homogenous mass.

VIVA- QUESTIONS

1. ***What do you mean by semi solid dosage form?***
2. ***What are advantages and disadvantages of semi solid dosage form?***
3. ***What are the different types of semi solid dosage form?***
4. ***What are the commonly used excipients in semi solid dosage form?***
5. ***What are the storage conditions of semi solid dosage form?***
6. ***Which type of base is used in preparation of sulphur ointment?***
7. ***What is use of sulphur ointment?***

CHAPTER TWENTY-THREE

EXPERIMENT 23

AIM- To prepare non staining iodine with methyl salicylate.

MATERIALS REQUIRED- Beaker, stirrer, China dish, pipette, measuring cylinder.

FORMULA

INGRIDIENTS	QUANTITY USED	ROLE OF INGREDIENT
Iodine	2.5g	Counter irritant
Oleic acid	2.0ml	Source of unsaturated fatty acid
Castor oil	2.5ml	Source of unsaturated fatty acid
Methyl Salicylate	12.0 ml	Anti- inflammatory
Soft paraffin q.s. ad	50 g	Ointment base

Composition of Non staining iodine with methyl salicylate

THEORY

Iodex, a trusted pain relief brand helps provide a warning action upon massage that helps in inflammation and provides effective relief from every type of Body pain. They are also used for iodine deficiency, antiseptic.

PROCEDURE

1. Iodine is dissolved in oleic acid at room temperature by simply stirring in a beaker.
2. Heat the above solution on water bath at 50°C with occasional stirring until brown colour disappear and replaced by greenish black colour.
3. Sufficient quantity of paraffin is added (previously heated), stir slowly and cool to solidify and add castor oil. Add methyl salicylate to Semi- solid preparation.
4. Pack in a tightly closed wide mouth bottle.

NON-STAINING IODINE METHYL SALICYLATE

FORMULA- Iodine (2.5g), oleic acid (2g), castor oil (2.5ml), methyl salicylate (12ml), and soft paraffin q.s. 50 g

USES- Relief from back acne and muscle strain.

CATEGORY- counter-irritant

DIRECTION- for external use only. Do not apply on broken skin.

MFG Date- 25 Aug 2017

EXP Date- 24 Aug 2018

MFG BY- M.P Pharmaceutic Pvt. Ltd.

BATCH NO- 111AP47

MFG. LICENSE NO- 191999

MRP- ₹70/-

Enter Caption

CATEGORY

Counter irritant.

STORAGE

Store in cool place.

DIRECTION

For external use only.

USES

Provides long lasting relief from back ache, waist acne, muscle strain, sprain

RESULT

Non- staining iodine with methyl salicylate was prepared.

VIVA- QUESTIONS

1. ***Define ointments, cream, paste and jellies.***
2. ***What is the use of oleic acid in non- staining iodine with methyl salicylate.***
3. ***What do you mean by counter irritant?***
4. ***What is mechanism of penetration of drug across dermal area?***
5. ***What are the uses of non- staining iodine with methyl salicylate?***

CHAPTER TWENTY-FOUR

EXPERIMENT 24

AIM-To prepare and supply iodine gargle.

MATERIAL REQUIRED- Iodine, purified water, beaker, measuring cylinder, stirrer

FORMULA-

Povidone iodine- 1gm

Purified water- q.s. or 1000ml

THEORY-

Gargles are aqueous solutions used to treat or prevent throat infection which are usually available in concentrated form with direction for dilution with warm water before use. Gargles may be used to give symptomatic relief and antiseptic effect. Many gargles are diluted with water prior their use. They are intended to bring the medicament in contact with mucus surface of throat.

PROCEDURE-

1. Weighed 1gm of povidone iodine and transfer it to 1000ml measuring cylinder.
2. Then added boiled and cooled purified water and was stirred until povidone iodine was completely dissolved.
3. The preparation was transferred into alkaline free amber coloured fused glass bottles, capped, labelled, and submitted.

IODINE GARGLE

FORMULA- Povidone iodine- 1gm, purified water- q.s. or 1000ml

STORAGE- Stored in well closed container in a cool, dry, and ventilated area in tightly sealed container.

MFG Date- 20/10/17

EXP Date- 19/ 10/18

Batch No- A1P99

MFG By- PM Pharmaceutical Pvt Ltd.

MFG License- 99849

MRP- Rs. 161

Iodine Gargle Label

DIRECTION

'Diluted with an equal volume of warm water'

'For external use only'

'Not to be swallowed in large amounts'

CATEGORY

Topical antibacterial and antifungal

STORAGE

Stored in well closed container in a cool, dry, and ventilated area in tightly sealed container.

RESULT

Iodine gargle was successfully prepared and dispensed.

VIVA- QUESTIONS

1. ***Define gargles and mouthwashes.***
2. ***What is the direction of use for gargles and mouthwashes?***
3. ***What is use of povidone iodine gargle?***
4. ***What is method of preparation for povidone iodine gargle?***

CHAPTER TWENTY-FIVE

EXPERIMENT 25

AIM- To prepare and submit 10ml of chlorohexidine mouthwash.

MATERIAL REQUIRED- Sodium fluoride, Chlorohexidine gluconate, Zinc chloride, Purified water, beaker, stirrer, measuring cylinder

FORMULA-

SNo.	INGREDIENTS	QUANTITY USED
1.	Chlorohexidine gluconate	0.2gm
2.	Sodium fluoride	0.05gm
3.	Zinc chloride	0.09gm
4.	Purified water	100ml

Composition of Chlorohexidine Mouthwash

THEORY-

Mouthwashes are aqueous solutions, often in concentrated form, containing one or more active ingredients and excipients. Mouthwashes in concentrated form need to be diluted as per directions on the label. A pH of 5-9.5appears to be safe range with 6.5- 7 being optimum for liquids for oral use.

Mouthwashes are classified as:

Therapeutic mouthwashes

These are used for specific problem in oral cavity.

E.g., mouthwashes containing antibacterial, fluoride or astringent agent.

Cosmetic mouthwashes

These are formulated to reduce bad breath through the use of antimicrobial agents or flavouring agents.

Chlorohexidine gluconate is disinfectant and topical anti- infective agent to prevent oral plaque. It is antimicrobial and bactericidal. Sodium fluoride is used to prevent cavities. It makes teeth more resistant to decay caused by acid and bacteria. Zinc chloride is necessary trace element in the diet, forming an essential part of enzymes and playing an important role in protein synthesis and in cell division. Chlorohexidine gluconate is a broad-spectrum antibacterial compound. Its commonly used in dentistry in the treatment of gum disease. One of its beneficial characteristics is that its strongly absorbed to oral surfaces. After rinsing approximately 30% of compound is retained in the user's mouth, creating a reservoir for sustained antibacterial activity. Its antimicrobial effects also help to create a reduction in breath odour over the long- term. Zinc is the metal of choice for rinses used to treat bad breath.

PROCEDURE-

1. Weighed quantity of chlorohexidine gluconate, sodium fluoride and zinc chloride were dissolved in $3/4^{th}$ quantity of purified water and stirred.
2. The final volume is adjusted with purified water.

3. The preparation was then transferred to well closed container, labelled, and submitted.

CHLOROHEXIDINE MOUTHWASH

FORMULA- Sodium fluoride (0.05gm),
Chlorohexidine gluconate (0.2gm),
Zinc chloride (0.9gm), Purified water (100ml)

USES- Treatment and prevention of gingivitis and maintenance of oral hygiene.

DIRECTION- Shake well before use

MFG Date- 20/10/17
EXP Date- 19/ 10/18
Batch No- A1P99
MFG By- PM Pharmaceutical Pvt Ltd.
MFG License- 99849
MRP- Rs. 118

WARNING- Not to be swallowed

Chlorohexidine Mouthwash Label

CATEGORY

Treatment and prevention of gingivitis and maintenance of oral hygiene.

DIRECTION-

- For treatment and prevention, swish in mouth for one minute.
- Do not wash mouth, eat or drink thereafter for 20 minutes.
- For prolonged use, take 1:1 dilution of sensoseal mouthwash with plain water.
- Shake well before use
- For dental use only

WARNING

Not to be swallowed.

STORAGE

Store in a cool, dry, and dark place.

RESULT

10ml of chlorohexidine mouthwash was prepared and dispensed.

VIVA- QUESTIONS

1. *What is the use of chlorohexidine mouthwash?*
2. *What is the direction of use for chlorohexidine mouthwash?*
3. *What is the use of chlorohexidine mouthwash?*
4. *What is the warning for chlorohexidine mouthwash?*
5. *Classify mouthwashes.*

CHAPTER TWENTY-SIX

EXPERIMENT 26

AIM- To prepare and dispense 50 ml of Paracetamol Paediatric Elixir .

MATERIAL REQUIRED- paracetamol, ethanol, propylene glycol, chloroform spirit, invert sugar, amaranth solution, glycerol, beaker, glass rod and measuring cylinder.

FORMULA-

S No.	INGREDIENTS	QUANTITY PRESCRIBED	QUANTITY USED
1.	Paracetamol	2.5gm	0.05gm
2.	Sucrose	667gm	20.01gm
3.	Distilled water	1000ml	30ml
4.	Preservatives	q.s.	q.s.

Composition of Paracetamol Paediatric Elixir

THEORY-

Elixirs are clear, flavoured, sweetened, hydro alcoholic liquid preparations for oral administration. The percentage of alcohol varies from 4 to 40% in this elixir. Paracetamol is used as antipyretic and analgesic.

Propylene glycol, ethanol and glycerol, there are all vehicles and co-solvents to increase the solubility of poorly soluble ingredients.

Chloroform spirit acts as a preservative.

Invert syrup acts as a sweetening agent.

Antipyretics reduce fever whereas analgesics help in reducing pain.

PROCEDURE-

1. Dissolve paracetamol in a mixture of ethanol (96%), propylene glycol and chloroform spirit.
2. The amount of alcohol is not sufficient to dissolve prescribed quantity of paracetamol, but due to combination of solvents, its solubility is enhanced.
3. Add rest of the ingredients with constant stirring, glycerol, and distilled water to produced 50 ml.

Rx

PARACETAMOL PAEDIATRIC ELIXIR IP 50ml

BABYLIX ELIXIR

EACH 5ml CONTAINES 125 mg OF PARACETAMOL

DOSAGE: AS DIRECTED BY PAEDIATRICIAN

STORE PROTECTED FROM LIGHT IN ORIGINAL CONATINER

MFD BY-

VG PHARMA

320, SOLAN INDUSTRIAL AREA, HIMACHAL PRADESH, INDIA

REG NO- 1247892

INGREDIENTS- ETHANOL (5ml), PROPYLENE GLYCOL (5ml), PARACETAMOL (1.2gm), CHLOROFORM SPIRIT (1ml), INVERT SYRUP (15ml), AMARANTH SOLUTION (10ml), GLYCEROL (q.s.), PURIFIED WATER (q.s., 50ml)

B. NO.- XP24322

MFG.D- 22/09/2022

EXP.D- 21/09/2022

MRP- Rs.100.00

INCL. ALL TAXES

Enter Caption

DOSE- Each 5ml contains 125 mg of paracetamol.
DIRECTION- For internal use only.
USE- Antipyretic and analgesic.
STORAGE- It should be protected from light.
ALCOHOL CONCENTRATION- 10 to 12% v/v.
RESULT- 50 ml of paediatric paracetamol elixir was prepared and dispensed.
VIVA- QUESTIONS

1. *What is elixir?*
2. *What is use of chloroform spirit in elixir?*
3. *What is role of propylene glycol in elixir?*
4. *What is concentration of alcohol in elixir?*
5. *What is use of elixir?*

9 798888 055717

Printed by Libri Plureos GmbH in Hamburg,
Germany